ii

The last days

Of

ALZHEIMER'S
DEMENTIA

The last days

Of

ALZHEIMER'S DEMENTIA

Summary of the Bredesen protocol

Precious C. Godson

Andy Iyama

Judy Skub

.

Dedicated to Alzheimer's patient all over the world

CONTENTS

❖ Chapter One   ------------------- Pg. 1
   Introduction to Dementia

❖ Chapter Two   -------------------Pg. 7
   Causes of dementia

❖ Chapter Three -------------------Pg. 12
   Dementia risk and prevention

❖ Chapter Four   -------------------Pg. 16
   Alzheimer's disease

❖ Chapter five   -------------------Pg. 20
   Stages and signs of Alzheimer's disease

❖ Chapter six   -------------------Pg. 31
   Causes of Alzheimer's

❖ Chapter seven -------------------Pg. 36
   Risk factors for Alzheimer's

❖ Chapter eight   -------------------Pg. 39
   Summary of the Bredesen protocol

❖ Chapter nine   -------------------Pg. 87
   Things You Must Know About Alzheimer's disease

To all fellow research-door researchers, your tireless effort in seeing to the progress and publication of this book is highly appreciated.

This piece is for educational use only, and not a doctor's prescription. It is not an advertisement for any product. Please consult your doctor to ascertain the best medical measures to take.

Chapter One
INTRODUCTION TO
dementia

Meaning of Dementia: Dementia regarded to be the most common term used to describe the decline in mental ability is strong enough to interfere with daily life. Example of such is memory loss. The most common type of dementia is Alzheimer – you will know more in the course of this study.

One thing to note here is that Dementia is not specifically a disease. It is a term that is widely used to describe various symptoms that is associated with a decline in memory (or other activities that involves thinking which is severe enough to reduce someone's performance while doing the day's activities. Before we go further, Alzheimer's disease accounts for about 60.1 – 80% of cases. While the second most common type of dementia is vascular dementia – which normally occurs after a stroke.

However, there are conditions that can have symptoms related to dementia including some that are irreversible, such as thyroid problems and deficiencies in a vitamin.

Dementia is often incorrectly believed to a serious mental decline been a normal part of aging – senile dementia.

Types of Dementia

The different types of dementia include:
• Alzheimer's
• Vascular dementia
• Dementia with Lewy bodies
• Mixed dementia
• Parkinson's disease
• Front-temporal dementia

- Creutzfeldt-Jakob disease
- Normal pressure hydrocephalus
- Huntington's disease
- Wernicke-Korsakoff Syndrome
- Progressive supranuclear palsy (PSP)

Symptoms of Dementia

Symptoms of dementia vary greatly from one to another. The following are the symptoms:

- Memory loss.
- A loss in communication and language.
- A decline in the ability to focus and pay attention.
- A decline in reasoning and judgment.
- Decline in visual perception

Before we consider dementia as being present in any issue that involves the brain, at least two of the core mental functions must be significantly impaired.

An individual with dementia may have problems with short-term memory, such as planning and preparing meals, remembering appointments, keeping track of wallet, paying bills etc.

Studies have shown that many dementias are progressive, which means that the symptoms start slowly and gets worse gradually. Anyone experiencing memory difficulties or in thinking skills should not be ignored. He/she is to see a doctor in other to determine the cause. Meeting a professional might detect a treatable condition that is not dementia, and if it suggests dementia after evaluation, early diagnosis allows a person to get the maximum benefit from available treatments.

Chapter Two

Causes of Dementia

The major cause of Dementia is brain cells damage. This damage interferes with the ability of the brain cells to communicate with each other. Therefore, this can affect thinking, feelings, and behavior, because they are not communicating normally.

Most changes that cause brain damage are permanent and can grow worse over time. However, the conditions mentioned below most times leads to memory loss

- Depression
- Thyroid problems.
- Vitamins deficiencies.
- Excess use of alcohol.
- Medication side effects.

These conditions require proper treatment.

The brain as the power function of the human anatomy has many distinct regions, responsible for various functions – such as movement, memory, judgment. Because of this, when cells in a particular region are damaged, they cannot carry out their functions normally.

There are different types of dementia associated with a particular type of brain cell damage in a particular region.

DIAGNOSIS

Dementia can be determined through physical examination, medical history, characteristic changes in thinking and laboratory tests.

It can as well be determined with a high level of certainty. In all these, it is difficult to ascertain the exact type of dementia that an individual has because the symptoms and brain changes of different dementias overlap – which then makes a doctor to diagnose dementia but will not be capable to specify the exact type.

The specialist best suitable for dementia diagnosis is a neurologist or gero-psychologist.

Chapter Three

Dementia risk and prevention

There are two major risk factors that can never change, which are age and genetics. However, other risk factors considered as active risk factors also pose as a threat. They include the following:

Diet: The food we eat has a tremendous impact on our body system – especially the brain (this implies that healthy brain affects the heart healthily too). Therefore, our eating goes a long way. Meals that have proven effective is the Mediterranean diet, which includes fruits and vegetables, fish and shellfish, nuts, olive oil, healthy fats, little red meat, and grains. This diet, when combined in the right proportion, may help protect the heart.

Physical exercise: Studies have proved that exercise may help increase the flow of blood and oxygen to the brain. This thereby lowers the risk of some kinds of dementia making regular exercise beneficial to the brain.

Cardiovascular risk factors: The brain is said to be nourished by one of the body's richest networks of blood vessels, therefore whatever damages the blood vessels in any part of the body, is capable of damaging blood vessels in the brain, thereby depriving brain cells of vital food and oxygen. This will now lead us to say that blood vessel changes in the brain have connection with vascular dementia. These changes may interact to cause faster decline or more impairments.

Chapter Four

Alzheimer's disease

Understanding the basic concept of dementia now leads us into Alzheimer's dementia.

This is the most common form of dementia that causes problems with memory, thinking, and behavior. Symptoms of Alzheimer's develop gradually, get worse over time, and become very dangerous because of its interference to one's daily activity.

As a form of dementia, Alzheimer disease accounts for about 60 – 80% cases. Like most persons do tag Alzheimer as a form of dementia is not normally associated with aging, though this is the greatest risk factor – increase in age – and those majorly diagnose with the disease are 65yrs and older. About 5% of people with the disease have early onset Alzheimer's – younger-onset which will be discussed in our further studies – and it often appears when someone in their 40s or 50s.

It is a progressive disease because it worsens over time. Dementia symptoms worsen gradually over a number of years. Therefore, at the onset, memory loss is mild which later becomes worse at the late stage whereby the individual finds it difficult – a loss in the ability – to carry on a conversation and respond to the environment.

Research studies have proven that Alzheimer disease is the sixth leading cause of death in the United States and it has no cure, but treatments for the symptoms are available. Though these treatments cannot stop Alzheimer's from progressing, they can only slow the worsening symptoms and improve the quality of life.

Chapter Five
STAGES AND SIGNS OF ALZHEIMER

As our faces are different, so is the difference in the symptoms of Alzheimer's. It varies from one individual to another. Barry Reisberg, M.D., developed a seven framework of Alzheimer's disease. We can discuss these stages as follows.

- No impairment
- Very mild decline
- Mild decline
- Moderate decline
- Moderately severe decline
- Severe decline
- Very severe decline

Stage 1: No impairment

At this stage, the person does not experience any memory loss/problems.

The person does not show any sign/symptom of dementia when conversing with a medical professional. This stage is also termed "normal function"

Stage 2: Very mild decline

At this stage, the person experiences very mild cognitive decline – early signs of Alzheimer's. Therefore, affected individual may feel as if he or she is having memory lapses – that is, forgetting familiar words or the location of everyday objects. This means that we cannot detect symptoms of dementia during a medical checkup or by friends, family, or co-workers.

Stage 3: Mild decline: Mild cognitive decline occurs when friends, family, and co-workers begin to notice difficulties. At this point, a medical professional can detect the symptoms of dementia. In some cases, though not all, we can identify individuals suffering from dementia with these symptoms and they include:

- Noticeable problems coming up with the right word/name
- Forgetting the material that one has just read
- Misplacing/losing an object that is valuable
- Noticeable greater difficulty performing tasks at work or in social settings
- Increasing trouble with organizing or planning

Stage 4: Moderate decline

Moderate cognitive decline is when a medical professional would be able to detect clear symptoms in difficult areas like

- Becoming moody or withdrawn
- Forgetfulness about one's personal history
- Greater difficulty in carrying out complex tasks such as paying bills.
- Forgetting recent events
- Impaired ability in performing complex mental arithmetic

Stage 5: Moderate-severe decline

During moderate-severe cognitive decline, individuals would begin to need help while carrying-out day-day activities because gaps in memory and thinking are noticeable. Those with Alzheimer's disease at this stage may experience the following:

- Unable to recall personal address or high school attended.
- Confused about what day it is or where they are
- They still remember significant details about themselves and their families
- Difficulty in choosing proper clothing for the season or occasion
- Trouble with less challenging mental arithmetic
- Require no assistance with eating or using the toilet

Stage 6: Severe decline

According to what we have explained earlier, Alzheimer's is progressive. At this stage of severe cognitive decline, memory continues to grow worse thereby enhancing personality changes where those affected need extensive help with daily activities. Characteristics of people that fall into this stage are as follows.

- They may remember their own names but finds it difficult to remember personal history.
- They may lose awareness of recent experiences including their surroundings.
- They may be able to distinguish faces but a difficulty in remembering the names of their caregiver/spouse.
- They may need help dressing properly and may/without,

supervision makes mistakes such as putting pajamas.

- They tend to wander away or become lost.
- They tend to experience major behavioral changes.

Stage 7: Very severe decline

This is termed the final stage of the disease because affected individuals lose the ability to carry on a conversation, respond to their surrounding environment and to control movement. They cannot do things on their own, therefore needs help when carrying daily activities, such as using the toilet or eating. Most times, they may lose the ability to smile or even sit without support. They become impaired in swallowing, their muscles grow rigid, and their reflexes become abnormal.

General Symptoms of Alzheimer's disease

At any stage of Alzheimer's dementia, there are many symptoms that will be noticed during diagnosis through the progression through the stages is monitored closely because it forms the basis with which it can be managed.

1. Impairments to: reasoning, complex tasking, exercising good judgment:
- Poor understanding of safety risks
- Unable to manage finances
- Inability to make good decisions
- Inability to plan sequential or complex activities.

2. Inability to remember and take-in new information, for example:

- Repetition of questions or conversations
- Often misplacement of personal belongings.
- Forgetting – unable to remember – events or appointments
- Getting lost on a familiar route or wandering.

3. Impaired Visuospatial abilities (though not due to eyesight problems):

- Unable to recognize faces, common objects or to find objects in direct view
- Unable to operate simple implements or orient clothing to the body.

4. Impairment of reading, speaking and writing:

- Difficulty in thinking of common words while speaking.
- Speech, spelling, and writing errors.

5. Personality and behavioral changes, for instance:

- Loss of empathy.
- Compulsive, obsessive, or socially – public – unacceptable behavior.
- Agitation, less interest, motivation or initiative; apathy; social withdrawal which has to do with Out-of-character mood changes.

Chapter Six
CAUSES OF ALZHEIMER'S

Research proved that Alzheimer's dementia is a disease commonly caused by a combination of lifestyle, genetic and environmental factors. However, there is more research going on to ascertain the root cause of this disease, its effect on the brain is clear. Alzheimer's dementia damages and kills brain cells. When the brain is affected, it reduces the cells and there will be fewer connections among surviving cells.

As the disease starts progressing, more brain cells die, thereby causing brain shrinkage. When we subject the brain tissue under a microscope, two types of abnormalities being the hallmarks of Alzheimer's disease exists. They include:

- **Plaques:** These are clumps of a protein called beta-amyloid, which may damage brain cells in several ways, such as interfering with cell-to-cell communication. In Alzheimer's, the death of brain cells is not yet known but these plaques are seen to be a prime suspect because of the collection of clumps of protein.

- **Tangles:** Every nerve in our body system are linked to the brain, thereby making brain cells to depend on an internal transport and support system to carry essential materials and other nutrients throughout their long extensions. In addition, this system requires normal structure and functioning known as **Tau protein.** The threads of Tau protein twist into abnormal tangles inside the brain cells, which lead to failure of the transport system.

Chapter Seven
Risk factors for Alzheimer's

We are going to about the major risk factors known so far. These includes the following

Genetics & Family history: Genetic mechanisms of Alzheimer's among most families are unexplainable now. However, Apo lipoprotein E4 (ApoE4) is seen to be the strongest risk gene of the disease, though not everyone with this gene develops Alzheimer's.

Alzheimer's disease can be hereditary, if a/the first-degree relative –especially the parents or siblings – is/are affected by the disease. Scientists have proven that this can occur when there is gene mutation, but less than 5% accounts to cause Alzheimer's dementia.

Sex: Women are prone to infection by Alzheimer's dementia than men because they live longer.

Down syndrome: It appears that about 10 – 20yrs earlier in people with Down syndrome than others do. This is so because a gene in the extra chromosome that causes Down syndrome increases the risk of Alzheimer's disease.

Age: Age is the greatest known risk factor for Alzheimer's dementia. We are not talking about normal aging, rather the risk increases as one clocks 65yrs and beyond. The rate of dementia doubles every decade after 60yrs.

Head trauma of the past: This applies to those who havc had severe head trauma.

There are other lifestyle contributors to Alzheimer's, and they can enhance the development of heart disease. They include

- Poorly controlled type 2 diabetes
- High blood cholesterol
- High blood pressure
- Obesity
- Lack of exercise
- Lacking fruits and vegetables in our diets

Therefore, whatever that poses a risk factor for heart disease is also a threat to develop into Alzheimer's disease and increase the risk of vascular dementia.

Chapter Eight

Summary of the Bredesen Protocol

(Compiled by Andy Iyama)

The Bredesen protocol in over 250 subjects proved effectively to reverse cognitive decline in neurodegenerative diseases such as Alzheimer's disease and Dementia.

Dr. Dale Bredesen and his team at MPI Cognition developed the Bredesen Protocol. MEND protocol was its former name, but now is called ReCODE. The overall goal of this protocol is to fix the following (which in turn reverses cognitive decline and helps with Alzheimer's and Dementia):

- Insulin resistance
- Inflammation/infections
- The hormone, nutrient, and trophic factor optimization.

- Toxins (chemical, biological, and physical)
- Restoration and protection of lost (or dysfunctional) synapses

Protocols like this may never reach global recognition or even FDA consideration for further evaluation. The problem with most FDA-based studies is that they only look at one aspect of the disease - X causes Y. Unfortunately, an Alzheimer's disease is complex and there are many root causes of it.

Most medical practitioners use advanced protocol, but ReCODE is a great place for someone in the early stages of Alzheimer's or Dementia to start.

Amyloid Plaques

Amyloid Precursor Protein: Amyloid precursor protein (APP) is naturally occurring in the brain and it depends on how it is cut by either netrin-1 or other molecules. It can either turn into-

1. Something healthy for the brain (such as sAPPα and αCTF)

   OR

2. Something toxic such as amyloid-beta (as well as Jcasp and C31)

If APP is to produce amyloid-beta, then amyloid-beta can continue to cut APP into more amyloid-beta plaques. This creates a positive feedback loop, thus creating more and more amyloid-beta plaques in the brain, instead of creating healthy molecules for the brain

This positive feedback loop creates a destructive effect on the synapses, instead of a plastic (protective) response.

Amyloid-Beta Plaque: The dogma behind amyloid plaque – the sticky plaque that builds up in the brain of Alzheimer's patients – as the main evil in Alzheimer's disease is actually incorrect. In fact, it may be protective in the following ways:

- Acts as an anti-microbial
- Binds to toxins (like heavy metals)
- Protects against inflammation

For example, one gets a bullet wound, would he/she just patch up the wound and not remove the bullet.

No, he/she would treat the underlying problems (remove the bullet) and replace the blood loss. The Bredesen Protocol first targets the underlying problem.

Types of Alzheimer's Dementia

There are three types of Alzheimer's disease described in the ReCODE protocol. They include the following.

1. Inflammation: Anything that causes inflammation to the brain (low chronic inflammation can do this as well) can contribute to Alzheimer's disease:

- AGEs
- ApoE4 (and ApoE3)
- Diet High in Lectins
- Imbalances in fatty acids (omegas)
- Infections
- Insulin Resistance
- Leaky Gut or Leaky Blood-Brain Barrier
- Neuroinflammation
- Toxins (including metals)

1.5 Glycotoxic: Glycotoxicity comes from an imbalance of glucose/insulin usage in the brain.

The pancreas produces Insulin-Degrading Enzyme (IDE, the enzyme that breaks down insulin) to break down amyloid beta.

If IDE used up by a diet rich in sugar – such as those with insulin resistance – break down of amyloid-beta will not be possible.

We regard this type of Alzheimer's to be 1.5 because it is a combination of Alzheimer's disease

1. inflammation and Alzheimer's disease
2. Trophic loss.

For example, having high amounts of glucose in the blood creates inflammation, and having improper usage of insulin, degrades insulin's ability to act as a neurotrophic – brain growth – promoter. Intranasal insulin may help with this type.

2. Metabolic/Trophins Loss

This type of Alzheimer's disease is usually caused by imbalances in the endocrine system (hormones) and nutrient depletion, as well as the neurotrophic loss (brain breaking down faster than it can regrow). These include:

- ApoE4
- Hormone Imbalances (Vitamin D, Sex and Neuro Steroids, Thyroid)
- Insulin Resistance
- Methylation Problems
- Mitochondrial Damage Neurotrophic Loss (atrophy in brain)
- Nutrient Depletion

3.Toxins: The toxin/infectious type of Alzheimer's disease are environmental caused by:

- ApoE3 (more common)
- Heavy Metals (including amalgams)
- Hormonal Imbalances
- HPA-Axis Imbalances
- Infections (such as mold, Lyme, HSV, active EBV, oral/nasal/gut dysbiosis)
- Low Zinc/high copper ratio
- Psychiatric disorders (correlation)
- Toxins (including pesticides, NSAIDS, PPIs, statins, and other drugs)

This usually occurs after the age of 80

Testing/Biomarkers

Note this is for educational purpose. Make sure you consult your doctor for proper checkup. In this section, we are going to talk about the tests to carryout. They are as follows.

Blood tests:

- Albumin/Globulin Ratio (A:G Ratio)
    - ○ ≥ 1.8
    - ○ >4.5 (albumin)
- Alpha-MSH
    - ○ 35 −81 pg/ml
- Arsenic
    - ○ <7 mcg/L
- Cadmium
    - ○ <2.5 mcg/L
- Calcium

- 8.5-10.5 mg/dl
- Cholesterol
  - 150
- Complement C4a
  - < 2830 ng/ml
- Copper
  - 90-110 mcg/dL
- Copper: Zinc Ratio
  - 0.8-1.2
- Cortisol (morning)
  - 10-18 mcg/dL
- DHEA
  - 350-430 (women) mcg/dL
  - 400-500 (men) mcg/dL
- Estradiol (Estrogen)
  - 50-250 pg/ml
- Folate
  - 10-25 ng/ml
- Glucose (fasting)
  - 70-90 mg/dL

- Glutathione
  - 5-5.5 micromolar
- HbA1C
  - ≤5.6%
- HDL
  - >50
- HLA-DR/DQ
  - Negative
- Hs-CRP
  - ≤0.9 ng/dL
- Il-6
  - ≤3 pg/ml
- Insulin (fasting)
  - ≤4.5 microIU/ml
- LDL-p
  - 700-1000
- Lead
  - <2 mcg/dL
- Leptin
  - 0.5-13.8 ng/mL (male)

- o 1.1-27.5 ng/mL (female)
- Mercury
  - o <5 mcg/L
- MMP9
  - o 85-332 ng/mL
- Omega 6:3 Ratio
  - o 0.5-3.0
- Osmolality
  - o 280-300 mosmol
- Oxidized LDL
  - o <60 U/l
- Pregnenolone
  - o 50-100 ng/dL
- Progesterone
  - o 1-20 ng/ml
- Potassium
  - o 4.5-5.5 mEq/L
- RBC Magnesium
  - o 5.2-6.5 mg/dL
- RBC Thiamine Pyrophosphate

- o 100-150 ng/ml
- sdLDL
  - o <20 mg/dL
- Selenium
  - o 110-150 ng/ml
- T3
  - o 3.2-4.2 pg/ml (free)
  - o <20 ng/dL (reverse)
- T4
  - o 1.3-1.8 ng/dL (free)
- TSH
  - o <2 microIU/ml
- Testosterone
  - o 500-1000 ng/dL (total)
  - o 6.5-15 ng/dL (free)
- TGF-β1
  - o < 2380 pg/ml
- TNF-alpha
  - o ≤6 pg/ml
- Triglycerides

- <150
- Vasopressin
  - 1.0-13.3 pg/ml
- VEGF
  - 31-86 pg/mL
- VIP
  - 23-63 pg/mL
- Vitamin B6
  - 60-100 mcg/L
- Vitamin B12 (MMA test can complement, but isn't a replacement)
  - 500-1500 pg/ml
- Vitamin C
  - 1.3-2.5 mg/dL
- Vitamin D
  - 50-80 ng/ml
- Vitamin E (as Alpha-Tocopherol)
  - 12 –20 mcg/ml
- Zinc

- 90-110 mcg/mL

It is also a good idea to test for leaky gut, leaky brain, and food sensitivities:

- Cyrex Array 2 – leaky gut
- Cyrex Array ¾ - food sensitivities and gluten intolerance
- Cyrex Array 5 – autoantibodies
- Cyrex Array 20 – leaky blood brain barrier

Infections can travel to the brain (via a leaky brain) through the nose, vagus nerve, or eye such as:

- Aspergillus
- CIRS
- Gingivitis
- Lyme (Borrelia)
- HSV

- Syphilis (neurosyphhilus)

This can also cause meningitis. It is advisable to use an organic acid test for mitochondrial function testing, use is advisable. A urine culture should be free of mycotoxins. No MicroBiome should have dysbiosis or infections. Perform Imaging with the following:

- PET (FDG-PET, Amyloid PET, or
- Tau PET) MRI with volumetrics (Neuroreader or NeuroQuant).

Body mass index (BMI) should be 18 – 25, waistline < 35 inches (women) or < 40 inches (men).

Here are some cognitive tests:

- MMSE (Mini-Mental State Examination)

- MoCA (Montreal Cognitive Assessment) - A normal MoCA score is 26 to 30
- SAGE (Self-Administered Gerocognitive Examination)

GENETICS: ApoE4 – epsilon – is the most common genetic variable for predicting Alzheimer's dementia. It preforms the following functions.

- It reduces the clearance of amyloid-beta plaques
- It regulates over 1,700 different genes (1/20 of human genome)
- It shuts down the gene that makes SirT1, which helps with gene regulation (resveratrol would help this)
- It activates NF-κB, thus promoting inflammation.

ApoE4 (about 14% of the population) is the worst, followed by ApoE3 (about 78%), then ApoE2 (about 8%) lesser than the rest.

It is also a good idea to check any mutations or polymorphisms in any of the following APP, PS1, PS2, CD33, TREM2, CR1, and NLRP1.

Treatment

Treatment is different for everyone, meaning not everybody must have the same treatment but simply goes like this:

1. Fixing the underlying cause (such as infections, toxin exposure, chronic inflammation)

2. Changing lifestyle in order to increase neurotrophic factors and proper autophagy
3. Using diet and treatments so as to restore biomes and insulin sensitivity in the brain/body
4. Optimizing hormones and other biomarkers using the following, bioidentical hormones, supplements, and herbs

Infections: Treat MARCoNs if positive. Also, inactivate/excrete pathogens using the following:

- IV glutathione
- Intranasal VIP
- Cruciferous foods

Here are some other useful tools to help remove infections or toxins:

- Activated charcoal
- Alpha lipoic acid
- Chitosan
- Chlorella
- Cholestyramine
- Guggul
- Manganese
- NFR2 activation
- Restore4life
- Sauna
- Vitamin B6
- Vitamin C
- Welchol
- Zinc Picolinate

LIFESTYLE: One cannot overlook this aspect. The following are life requirements for the ReCODE protocol that help reverse Alzheimer's disease

1. Sleep:
   a. 8-hrs of sleep/night (going to bed before midnight will also help)
   b. Avoid the use of blue light at night
   c. Avoid the use of EMFs at night

2. Brain stimulation:
   a. Engage yourself in brain training games
   b. Exercise regularly
   c. Increase neurotrophic factors (for example BDNF and NGF, also CNTF, GDNF, CDNF, and MANF is recommended)

3. Psychological

    a. For reduced atrophy, try to avoid stress

4. Oral hygiene

    a. Coconut pulling

    b. Brush and floss daily. Make it a habit

DIET: The ReCODE diet popularly called KETOFLEX 12/3. It has to do with being in ketosis, eating high amounts of fiber, eating within a 12-hr window, and stop eating at least 3-hrs before bed. The aim/goal is:

- To increase ketone bodies (such as acetoacetate, beta-hydroxybutyrate, and acetone)

- MCT oil (such as caprylic acid as the strongest form) is a must for ApoE4 and APOE until insulin sensitivity is restored, then switch to MUFAs and PUFAs

- Predominantly use lots of uncooked
  - Veggies
  - Fasting at least 12 hours/day
  - Stop eating 3 hours before bed
  - Increase insulin sensitivity

Foods: One is expected to eat the following frequently.

- Avocados
- Artichokes
- Beets
- Cilantro
- Cruciferous vegetables (such as cauliflower, broccoli/broccoli sprouts, various types of cabbage, kale, radishes, Brussels sprouts, turnips, watercress, kohlrabi, rutabaga, arugula, horseradish,

maca, rapini, daikon, wasabi, and
bok choy)
- Dandelions
- Garlic
- Ginger
- Grapefruit
- Jicama
- Kimchi
- Leafy greens (such as kale
  spinach, and lettuce)
- Leeks
- Lemons
- Mushrooms
- Olive oil
- Onions
- Pasture-raised eggs Resistant
  starches (such as sweet potatoes,
  rutabagas, parsnips, and green
  bananas)
- Sauerkraut

- Seaweed
- Tea (black and green)
- Wild-caught fish (SMASH fish such as salmon, mackerel, anchovies, sardines, and herring)

Now having known the foods to eat, we are going to look at foods we are not to eat frequently.

- Less coffee (e.g. Super coffee)
- Less grass-fed beef
- Less legumes (such as peas and beans)
- Less nightshades (such as eggplant, peppers, and tomatoes)
- Less Nontropical fruits (low glycemic, such as berries)
- Less pasture raised chicken

- Less starchy veggies (such as corn, peas, squash, but sweet potatoes are an exception)
- Less wine (1 glass/week)

In addition, here is a list food we are to avoid completely:

- Avoid dairy (occasional cheese or plain yogurt is okay, I recommend A2based dairy)
- Avoid fruits (high glycemic ones especially)
- Avoid gluten
- Avoid grains
- Avoid high mercury fish (such as tuna, shark, and swordfish)
- Avoid processed foods
- Avoid sugar and simple carbs (including loaves of bread,

wheat, rice, cookies, cakes, candies, sodas, etc.)

Most importantly, one also has note the following:

- Avoid overheating foods (as it creates AGEs)
- Fish is good, but do not do too much meat.
- Remove all Lectins. Just an advice
- If you do eat fruits, make sure they are rich in fiber and not as juice.
- Include lots of good fats in your diet (such as avocados, olive oil, MCT oil like caprylic acid and if non-Lectins sensitive then nuts and seeds oils are okay)
- Use digestive enzymes

MicroBiome

This includes prebiotics and probiotics:

- B. lactis (fermented dairy)
- B. longum (fermented veggies and dairy)
- L. acidophilus (fermented dairy)
- L. brevis (sauerkraut and pickles)
- L. plantarum (kimchi, sauerkraut and fermented veggies)
- Probiomax
- S. boulardi

If you have, any infections with biofilms you must take care of those as well (may use Bactroban/Mupirocin, SinuClenz, or Xlear).

For the nasal MicroBiome:

- Try Kimchi juice + nasal swab
- And Restore4Life

Insulin Resistance: Here are some supplements recommended for decreasing insulin resistance:

- Alpha lipoic acid
- Berberine
- Chromium picolinate
- Cinnamon
- Magnesium Glycinate
- Magnesium Threonate
- Metformin (drug)
- Zinc Picolinate

Supplements and Herbs

Supplements to the ReCODE program that help with cognition and inflammation are as follows:

- ALCAR
- Citicoline
- Coffee fruit extract
- DHA/EPA (fish oil or krill oil) R
- Nicotinamide riboside (combines well with resveratrol)
- Pantothenic acid (use B6/B12/folate if homocysteine $\geq$ 6)
- PQQ
- Resveratrol
- Ubiquinol
- Vitamin B1
- Vitamin C Vitamin D
- Vitamin E
- Vitamin K2
- Herbs on the ReCODE program that help with cognition and inflammation:
- Ashwagandha

- Bacopa
- Gotu Kola
- Guduchi
- Guggul (or activated charcoal)
- Lion's Mane
- Rhodiola
- Skullcap
- Triphala (Amalaki + Haritaki + Bibhitaki)

In addition, use pro-resolving mediators (SPM Active) such as resolvins, protectins, and maresins will also help against inflammation.

Mechanism of Action

Here are all the functions that the ReCODE protocol aims to accomplish:

> o Elevates α- cleavage
> o Elevates ADNP

- Elevates autophagy
- Improve axoplasmic transport
- Elevates BDNF
- Elevates cAMP
- Elevates GABA
- Elevates glutathione
- Elevates IDE
- Elevates insulin sensitivity
- Improve LTP
- Elevates NGF
- Elevates microglial clearance of Aβ
- Elevates netrin-1
- Elevates neprilysin
- Elevates PPAR-γ
- Elevates phagocytosis index
- Elevates PP2A
- Elevates resolvins
- Elevates SirT1

o Elevates synaptoblastic signaling

o Elevates telomere length

o Improve vascularization

o Elevates VIP

o Elevates vitamin D signaling

o Optimize all metals

o Reduce APPβ- cleavage

o Reduce caspase-6 cleavage

o Reduce caspase-3 cleavage

o Reduce γ- cleavage

o Reduce glial scarring

o Reduce homocysteine

o Reduce inflammation

o Reduce mTOR activation

o Reduce NF-κB

o Reduce phospho-tau

o Reduce oxidative damage and optimize ROS

o Reduce synaptoclastic signaling

Chapter Nine
THINGS YOU MUST KNOW ABOUT ALZHEIMER'S DISEASE

1. Dementia is not synonymous with Alzheimer's Disease:

The word dementia is an inclusive term for progressive brain syndromes that lead to a decline of brain functions such as memory, thinking, language, reasoning, and recognition abilities over time. Alzheimer's disease is the most common type of dementia and accounts for 60 to 80 percent of dementia cases. The most common sign of Alzheimer is memory loss, especially forgetting recently learned information. The typical changes that are age-related, such as forgetting names or appointments or getting confused about the day of the week, are usually a normal part of aging if they occur occasionally. However, if these episodes happen frequently and worsen over time, it is a warning sign of Alzheimer.

2. Alzheimer's can be life threatening:

The death of Alzheimer's patients usually occurs due to complications related to loss of critical brain functions. In the early stages of Alzheimer, patients suffer from forgetfulness and confusion. However, as the disease progresses, it becomes difficult for patients to move around and swallow food. This makes them particularly susceptible to infections such as pneumonia, which is the leading cause of death in persons with advanced Alzheimer's disease, urinary tract infections, and skin infections due to ulcers and bedsores. People with advanced Alzheimer's are also prone to falls, which can result in fatal head injuries or hip fractures. Alzheimer's patients also tend to wander away from home and get lost which puts them at risk of accidents and other dangerous situations.

3. Children are not exclusive

Alzheimer's is not be considered as a normal part of aging, but the most common form of Alzheimer's is late-onset Alzheimer's, which strikes older patients above the age of 65 years. According to estimates, dementia affects 5% of the population older than 65 with the rates increase with age. However, of all the people who have Alzheimer's disease, about 5 percent develop symptoms before age 65. While the exact cause of early-onset Alzheimer's is not precisely clear, rare genes, play a role too.

4. Genes are associated with Alzheimer's disease:

Genetics, lifestyle, and environmental factors affect the brain over time, which can lead to Alzheimer's dementia. Studies have revealed that certain genes can make one more susceptible to Alzheimer's disease. However, in order to establish the exact genetic disposition of Alzheimer's dementia, more research is required. Apolipoprotein E (APOE) is the most common gene associated with late-onset Alzheimer's disease. Therefore, having one APOE e4 gene increases the risk of Alzheimer's disease, with the risk becoming even higher with two APOE e4 genes - one gene inherited from each parent. Not everyone with either one or two APOE e4 genes develops Alzheimer's and in some cases, the disease occurs even in those with no APOE e4 genes.

Conclusion: Since we have seen

that Alzheimer's disease have no cure, it is advisable for one to engage in regular medical check-up. Though regular medical check-up is not the cure – do not get it twisted – it helps one to ascertain when something is wrong/better or good with the body system. Now during early diagnosis, the application of some researched medical therapies can go a long way in boosting one's health, and help build many antibodies that will help fight diseases.

In addition, to eradicate this disease completely from our world, one has to look into the preventive measures and work with them. Therefore, it is advisable that one reads the preventive measure once again. Avoid anything that

that can pose a risk factor for heart disease.

Together, today might be the end of Alzheimer's, so always consult your doctor for medical/professional advice.
Stay healthy, because Health is Wealth.

Notes:_____

_____

_____

_____

_____

_____

_____

_____

_____

_____

_____

_____

_____

_____

_____

_____

_____

_____

_____

_____

_____

_____

_____

_____

_____

_____

_____

_____

_____

_____

_____

_____

_____

_____

_____

_____

_____

_____

_____

_____

_____

_____

_____

_____

_____

_____

_____

_____

Made in the USA
Monee, IL
16 July 2023